Hèla Ben Jmaà
Rim Karray

Aortic aneurysms of inflammatory origin

Hèla Ben Jmaà
Rim Karray

Aortic aneurysms of inflammatory origin

Inflammatory aortic aneurysms

ScienciaScripts

Imprint

Cover image: www.ingimage.com

This book is a translation from the original published under ISBN 978-620-6-71936-6.

Publisher:
Sciencia Scripts
is a trademark of
Dodo Books Indian Ocean Ltd. and OmniScriptum S.R.L publishing group

120 High Road, East Finchley, London, N2 9ED, United Kingdom
Str. Armeneasca 28/1, office 1, Chisinau MD-2012, Republic of Moldova, Europe
Printed at: see last page
ISBN: 978-620-7-97950-9

Aortic aneurysms of inflammatory origin

I. Introduction :

Inflammatory aortitis is a disease characterized by infiltration of the aortic wall by inflammatory cells responsible for disorganization of the arterial tunics, leading to stenosis, thrombosis and/or vascular ectasia [1].

These complications may involve the aorta itself, but also its main branches [1].

Takayasu's disease, Horton's disease and Behçet's disease are the three main causes of inflammatory aortitis [1].

Positive diagnosis of inflammatory aortitis remains difficult, and its spontaneous evolution may be marked by the occurrence of several complications. The management of inflammatory aortitis presents a number of particularities compared to other forms of aortitis, and the prognosis is severe and life-threatening [1].

Their treatment has traditionally been based on conventional surgical management combined with prior corticosteroid therapy [1]. In recent years, endovascular treatment of these conditions has been developed, leading to a reduction in morbidity and mortality.

Takayasu disease is diagnosed according to the Ishikawa criteria [2].

The diagnosis of Behçet's disease is based on the criteria of the International Research Group for Behçet's Disease [3].

II. Etiologies :

The most common inflammatory vasculitides affecting the aorta are Horton's disease, Takayasu's disease and Behçet's disease [1].

Inflammatory involvement of the aorta has also been described in Buerger's disease, Kawasaki disease, Cogan syndrome, ankylosing spondylitis, sarcoidosis and systemic lupus erythematosus [4].

1- Takayasu disease:

Takayasu disease is an inflammatory arteritis of large and medium-caliber vessels, mainly affecting the aorta, its main dividing branches and the pulmonary arteries [5].

It often leads to stenosis, thrombosis and sometimes aneurysm formation [6].

2- Behçet's disease:

Behçet's disease is a systemic vasculitis that progresses in relapses. It combines oral-genital bipolar aphthosis, uveitis and systemic manifestations, notably cutaneous, articular, neurological and vascular (angio-Behçet) [1].

Angio-Behçet is dominated by thrombophlebitis [7]. Arterial involvement is rare, with acute lesions leading to aneurysms and arterial occlusions. It mainly affects the large trunks, notably the aorta, renal arteries, popliteal artery and pulmonary artery [8].

3- Horton's disease [1, 9]:

Horton's disease is an arteritis of the large and medium-caliber arteries. It preferentially affects the external carotid artery and its branches.

I- Epidemiology :

1- Takayasu disease:

Takayasu disease is a very rare form of arteritis [5]. The existence of a few large series including patients from Asia [10, 11], Africa [12], India [6] and Central America [13] has suggested that the prevalence of the disease may be higher in these ethnic groups.

Its peak incidence is typically in the second or third decade of life [5, 14]. However, paediatric forms and forms after the age of 40 are not exceptional [15, 16].

Aortic involvement is extremely frequent, occurring in 40-70% of patients with Takayasu disease [17]. L. Arnaud et al [5] reported on a single-center French series of 82 patients with Takayasu arteritis. In a North American study, the incidence was estimated at 2.6 cases/million/year [18].

2- Behçet's disease :

Behçet's disease is more common in the Mediterranean basin. It most often affects young adults between the ages of 20 and 40, with no cardiovascular risk factors [8]. Males are clearly more affected than females.

Arterial involvement affects 1-2% of patients [19]. Aneurysms are more frequent than occlusions. Aortic location is the most common, followed by iliac and femoral involvement.

Aneurysms of the abdominal sub-renal aorta are one of the most frequent localizations of arterial aneurysms in Behçet's disease. They may be associated with other aneurysmal locations, notably in the pulmonary arteries, femoral arteries and popliteal arteries. Aneurysms may be associated with arterial occlusions [20].

3- Horton's disease:

Horton's disease tends to affect elderly subjects, with a predominance of women [1, 21]. Aortic involvement is rare in Horton's disease [22].

Evans et al [23], in a retrospective study of 1,330 patients with Horton's disease, observed 3% aortic involvement.

In other historical retrospective series, aortic involvement has been described in 3 to 18% of cases [21].

III. Clinical study:

1- Takayasu disease:

Takayasu disease may present with general signs and/or polymorphous ischemic manifestations, reflecting the progressive formation of stenoses within the arterial tree [5]. It classically evolves in 2 phases: the systemic or pre-occlusive phase, and the occlusive phase [6].

During the systemic or pre-occlusive phase, non-specific general signs come to the fore.

Neurological manifestations reflect transient or cumulative ischemia of the central nervous system, associated with damage to the aortic arch and supra-aortic trunks [1, 5].

Ischemic damage to the celiac trunk and mesenteric arteries may be responsible for a picture of digestive angina, manifested by atypical or rhythmic abdominal pain.

The preferential location is the AMS, often affected over a long length [24].

Cutaneous manifestations such as :

- Nodular hypodermatitis

- Erythema nodosum

- Skin ulcerations

- Pyoderma gangrenosum

A diastolic murmur at the aortic focus is found in 5-30% of cases [5]. Physical examination reveals aortic insufficiency due to inflammatory damage to the ascending aorta and thickening of the aortic sigmoid [6].

It may also reveal sensory-motor deficits associated with ischemic stroke.

Fundus examination may reveal hypertensive retinopathy in patients with hypertension [25].

The most frequent dermatological signs are palpable subcutaneous nodules on the lower limbs. Erythema nodosum may also be indicative of the disease.

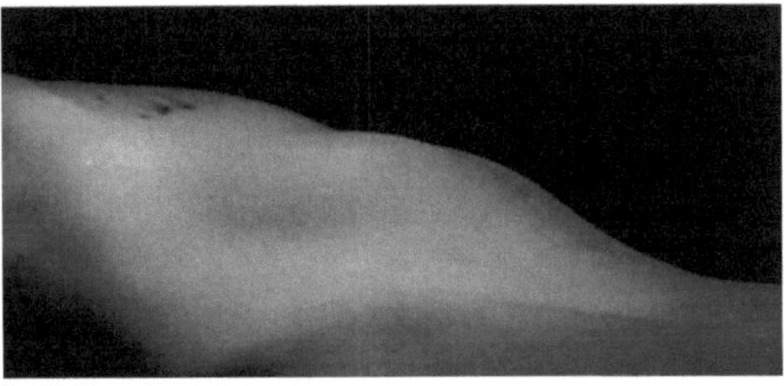

Figure 1: Photograph showing abdominal curvature.

2- Behçet's disease :

Moderate fever, isolated or associated with asthenia, may be noted at the start of an outbreak [26]. Recurrent mouth ulcers are usually the initial symptom that brings patients to the doctor. These are small, painful ulcerations of an isolated or multiple nature, occurring in flare-ups.

Other skin manifestations include :

- Erythema nodosum

- Pseudofolliculitis

- Acne nodules

- Migratory superficial thrombophlebitis

- Aspecific cutaneous hyperreactivity to attacks on the epithelium (whether from injections, superficial scratches or intradermal reactions to various antigens) [27].

Patients with eye lesions have variable symptoms including:

- Blurred vision

- Eye pain

- Photophobia

Joint involvement manifests as arthralgia. It often occurs early, and may precede other symptoms by several years [28].

Intermittent claudication-like pain in the lower limbs may indicate peripheral arterial or aortic damage.

Edema of a lower limb secondary to deep vein thrombosis may also reveal the disease.

Physical examination may also reveal abolition of one or more peripheral pulses, or a murmur in a vascular pathway. Arrhythmia on cardiac auscultation may complicate valvular disease.

Neurological damage can take various forms:

- A picture of meningitis or meningoencephalitis

- Damage to the cerebral parenchyma resulting in a picture of ischemic vascular accident, either permanent or transient: hemiplegia, aphasia...

- Cerebral venous thrombosis

Dermatological examination may reveal oral and genital aphthae, erythema nodosum, necrotic pseudofolliculitis, acneiform nodules and cutaneous hyperreactivity.

Anterior uveitis may be fleeting and clinically quiescent. It may only be visible on slit-lamp examination.

Aortic involvement may also be discovered by chance on clinical examination, ultrasound or abdominal CT scan.

3- Horton's disease: [29]

Horton's disease is characterized by :

- Angiodynia, particularly localized headaches of recent onset
- Clinical abnormalities of the temporal artery
- Ocular symptoms (fleeting amaurosis, diplopia)
- Claudication or trismus of the jaw
- Claudication of the tongue or on swallowing
- Respiratory signs (dry cough)
- A syndrome of the aortic arch, vertebral arteries and basilar trunk, which can lead to stroke-like symptoms (hemiplegia, hemiparesis, aphasia, etc.).
- A fever
- Arthralgia
- Myalgia

In the experience of the Amien and Rouen group [30], aortitis in Horton's disease is asymptomatic in 77% of cases, or may be revealed by dyspnea, abdominal pain or back pain. It is not usually accompanied by the presence of a pulsatile mass, aortic murmur or vascular murmur.

A poor clinical examination may reveal an abolition of the temporal pulse or a protruding, inflamed temporal artery. Symptoms of inflammatory aortitis depend on the vascular territory affected, the type of aortic involvement (aneurysmal or occlusive) and its location.

IV. Additional tests :

The major evolution is due to the use of current non-invasive imaging methods such as ultrasound-Doppler [31], angioscanner [32], MRI and MRI-angiography for the diagnosis and monitoring of the disease [33].

1- Biology :

There is no specific biological diagnostic marker for Takayasu disease, which is characterized by the presence of nonspecific general inflammatory signs [5, 34]. Increased sedimentation rate (ESR) and CRP are indicators of disease activity, while their decrease or even normalization is indicative of treatment efficacy or disease quiescence [35]. However, a normal VS does not rule out the disease, and vascular lesions may continue to evolve despite a normal VS [36].

In Behçet's disease, the following biological abnormalities may be observed:

- An often significant acceleration in sedimentation rate, generally > 50 in the first hour.

- Neutrophil-predominant hyperleukocytosis.

- Lymphopenia is common.

- An increase in alpha-2 globulins and gamma globulins, especially Ig M, Ig G and Ig A [37].

- Circulating immune complexes are found in 40-60% of cases, and their levels correlate with disease activity. Indeed, Ig G and Ig M immune complexes increase in parallel with disease activity, while Ig A complexes decrease [37, 38].

Horton's disease is not accompanied by any recognized antibodies, apart from anti-cardiolipin antibodies in less than a third of cases [29].

2- Chest X-ray:

A thoracic aortic aneurysm can be detected by an annual chest X-ray [39].

3- Echo-Doppler :

It allows precise study of the supra-aortic trunks, limb arteries, renal arteries, digestive arteries, and sometimes the abdominal aorta [40]. However, the study of abdominal vessels is possible, although technically hampered by the interposition of digestive structures [40].

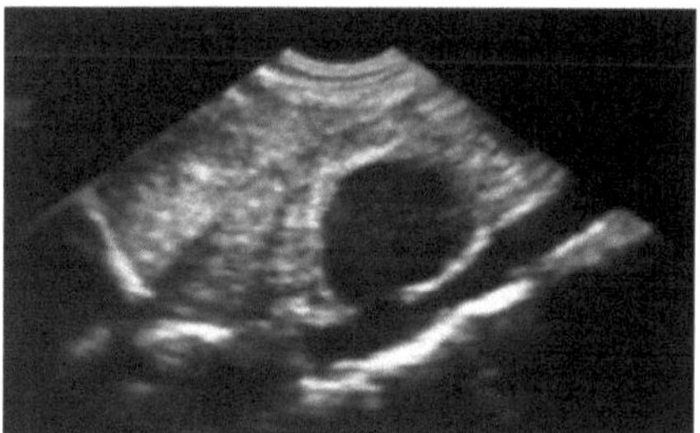

Figure 2: Doppler ultrasound showing a large saccular aneurysm of the abdominal aorta, probably fissured [40].

Abdominal Doppler ultrasonography shows the aortic aneurysm, specifying :

- Shape: fusiform or sacciform
- Dimensions: anteroposterior and transverse diameters
- Contents
- Its location above or below the kidney

- Its inflammatory nature: with a thickened and calcified aortic wall, and a homogeneous hypoechoic gangue draping the anterior wall of the aneurysm [41].

- The presence or absence of complications:

  - Fissuring, showing a peri-arterial hematoma visible as a faintly echogenic, often heterogeneous localized lamina.
  - Aneurysmal rupture, showing an anechoic, poorly circumscribed image of addition of the circulating channel, projecting outside the arterial contour [42].

However, ultrasound is less effective than CT and MRI for diagnosing the inflammatory nature of aneurysms and for diagnosing complications.

In Horton's disease, this technique can also visualize a hypoechoic halo in the superficial temporal artery or in large-caliber vessels [43, 44]. According to Shmidt et al [43], the presence of such a halo indicates inflammatory edema related to a specific localization of Horton's disease. However, this sign is far from constant [45, 46].

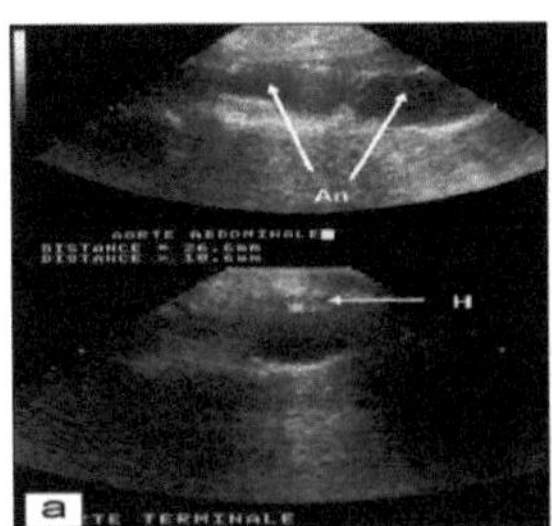

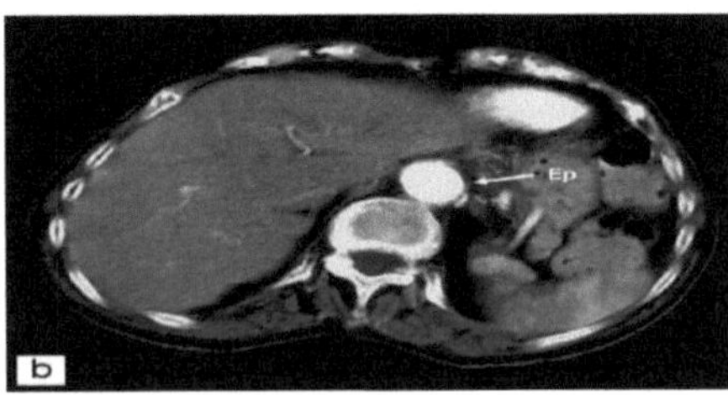

Figure 3: Abdominal aortic aneurysm in Horton's disease: double aneurysmal dilatation (An) in the abdominal aorta, associated with a hypoechoic periaortic halo (H) [47].

4- Angio-scanner [48]:

Angiography enables reliable angiographic images to be reconstructed non-invasively.

Given the frequent association of aortic lesions with occlusive or aneurysmal lesions of the visceral arteries or supra-aortic trunks in Takayasu disease, radiological exploration of the entire aorta and its collateral branches is necessary to establish therapeutic indications.

Angio-CT is more effective than echo-Doppler in diagnosing aortic aneurysms in Behçet's disease. It enables complete exploration of the aneurysm, specifying its morphology and extension, as well as exploration of the peri-aneurysmal inflammatory process.

The circulating component is intensely enhanced after injection of the contrast medium, the thrombus does not pick up the medium, and around the whole the periaurysmal fibrosis appears hyperdense with variable enhancement depending on the inflammatory stage.

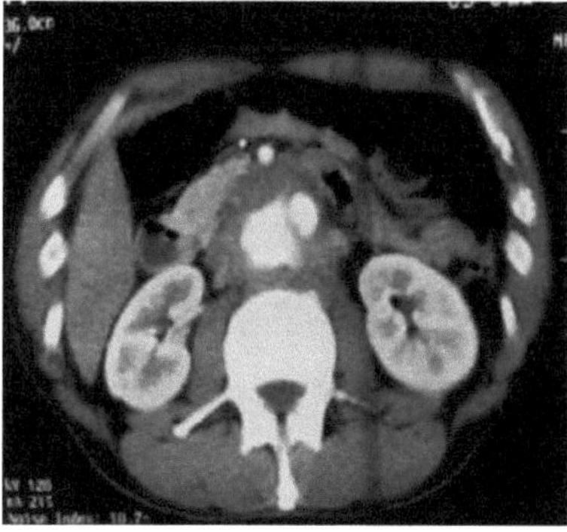

Figure 4: Abdominal CT scan with injections in axial section (A) and reconstruction (B), showing a saccular aneurysm of the abdominal sub-renal aorta in a patient with Behçet's disease [49].

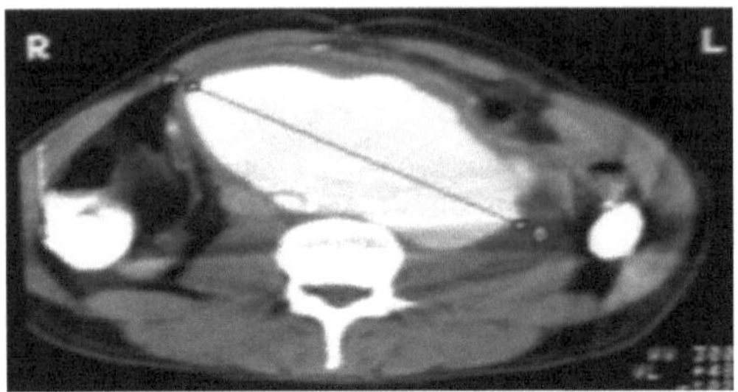

Figure 5: Scannographic section showing a 14 cm diameter saccular aneurysm in the abdominal sub-renal aorta in a patient with Behçet's disease.

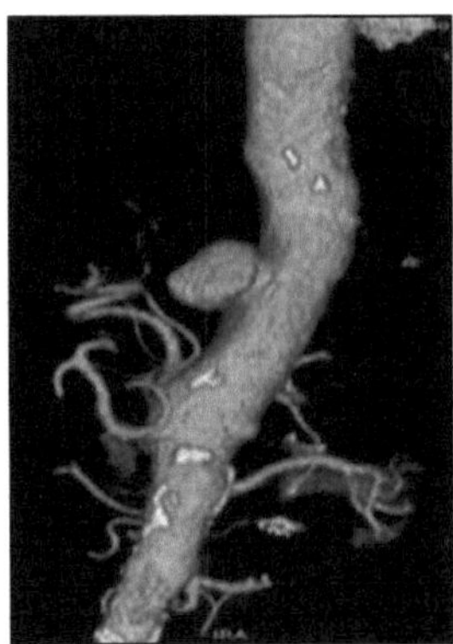

Figure 6: Partially thrombosed false aneurysm of the lateral aspect of the suprarenal abdominal aorta 5 cm from the ostium of the celiac trunk in a patient with Behçet's disease.

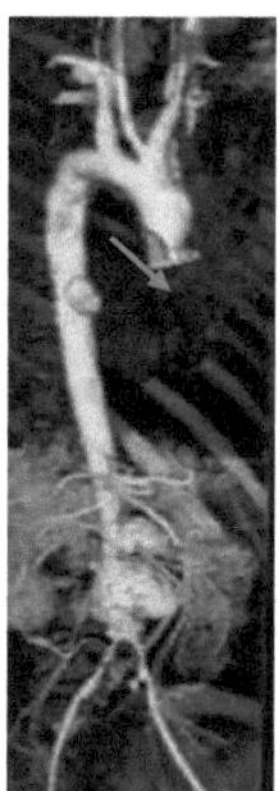

Figure 7: Two pseudoaneurysms: one of the descending thoracic aorta, the other of the aortic bifurcation in a patient with Behçet's disease.

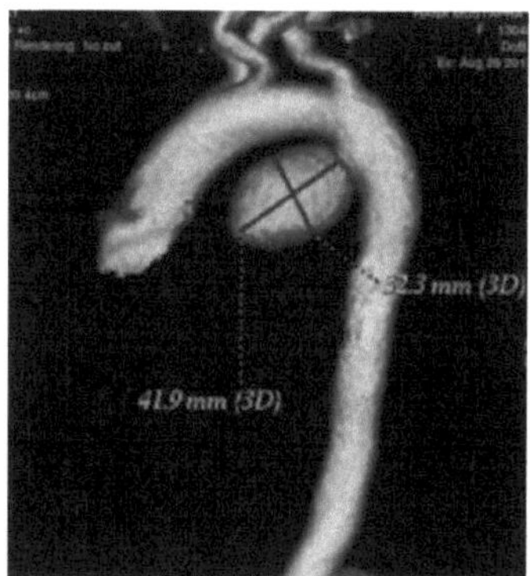

Figure 8: Angioscan reconstruction showing a pseudoaneurysm of the aortic arch in a patient with Behçet's disease.

The angio-scanner also highlights possible vascular lesions such as :

- stenoses
- occlusions
- aneurysms, which are rarer than stenosing lesions.

- the presence of concentric circumferential thickening of more than 2 mm of the arterial wall.

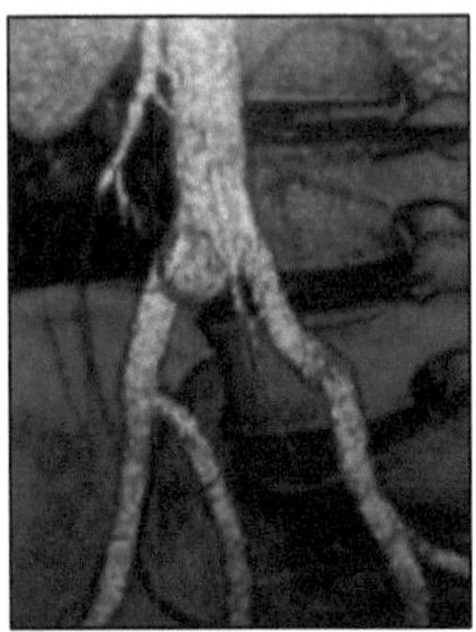

Figure 9: Angioscan showing an aortic bifurcation aneurysm in a patient with Takayasu disease [50].

Some authors have suggested that the presence of excessive aortic wall thickening (> 3 mm), early or late mural contrast or a low-attenuation ring within the arterial wall may reflect disease activity [51].

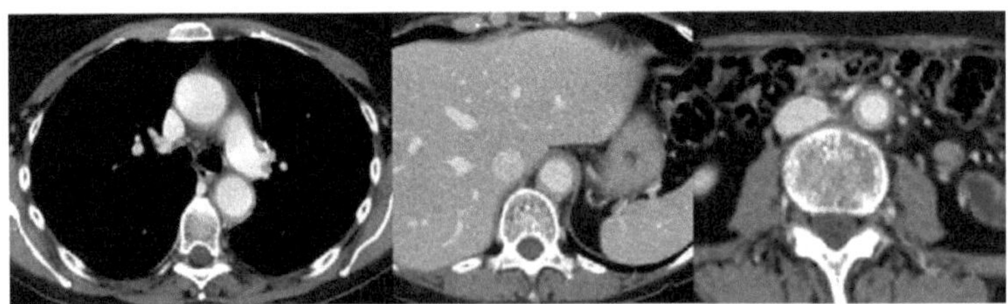

Figure 10: Thoracoabdominal CT scan with contrast injection showing regular thickening of the thoracic and abdominal aortic wall in Horton's aortitis [21].

5- Arteriography :

It enables a precise lesion assessment to be carried out prior to revascularization. Three types of lesions can be observed: stenoses, obliterations and aneurysms.

Arteriography clarifies the characteristics of the aneurysm, its location, fusiform or saccular type, and detects aortic collaterals arising from the aneurysmal sac (figure 11).

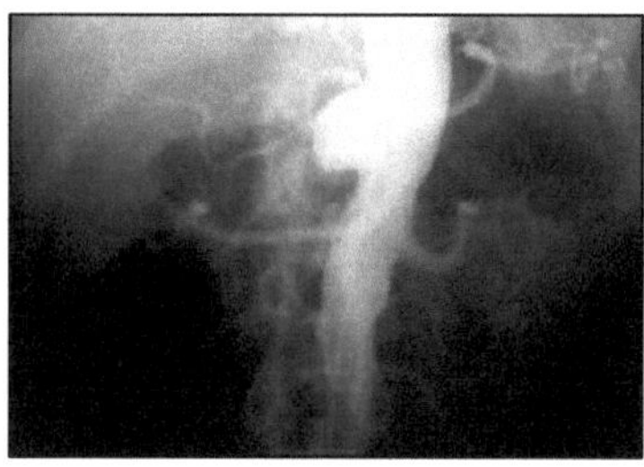

Figure 11: Angiography of the abdominal aorta showing a saccular aneurysm of the suprarenal aorta in a patient with Behçet's disease [52].

However, it is unreliable for assessing the size of the aneurysm, due to the possible existence of an aneurysmal thrombus, which leads to an underestimation of its true size.

In addition, the iatrogenic risk of arterial puncture must be taken into account, and angioscanning should be preferred for diagnosis.

In Horton's disease, the lesions found in the branches of the aorta are long, regular, fusiform stenoses, occlusions and ectasias. However, its invasive nature and advances in other imaging modalities limit its indications [21].

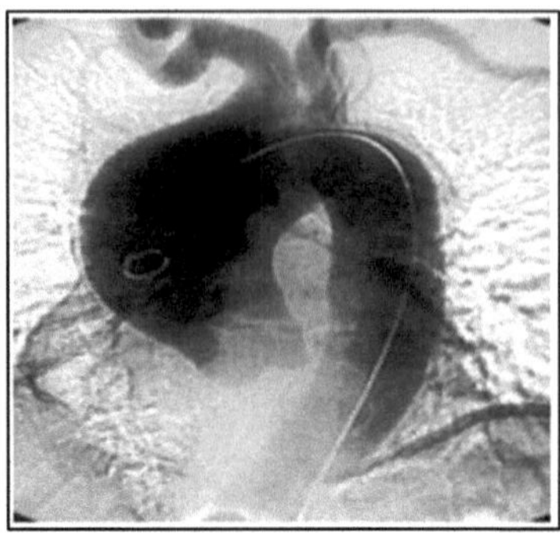

Figure 12: Aortography showing a fusiform aneurysm of the ascending aorta in Horton's disease [53].

6- Angio-MRI :

MRI angiography is a non-invasive, non-irradiating examination that visualizes the vascular wall and lumen.

The proposed activity criteria are the presence of diffuse, concentric arterial parietal thickening, reflecting the presence of arterial parietal inflammation, or even arterial stenoses [54].

MRI is as reliable as helical CT in diagnosing aneurysms and studying their various characteristics [41].

This is an excellent examination for diagnosing inflammatory aneurysms, showing a peri-arterial gangue with hypo T1 and variable T2 signal depending on the cellular reaction.

After gadolinium injection, enhancement of this peri-arterial mass is the rule, suggesting disease activity.

It has the advantage of excellent spatial resolution compared with PET, enabling both inflammation of the aortic wall and changes in the vascular lumen to be assessed. Concurrent study of the temporal arteries is possible [55].

Compared with PET, sensitivity for early diagnosis appears to be slightly lower [56, 57].

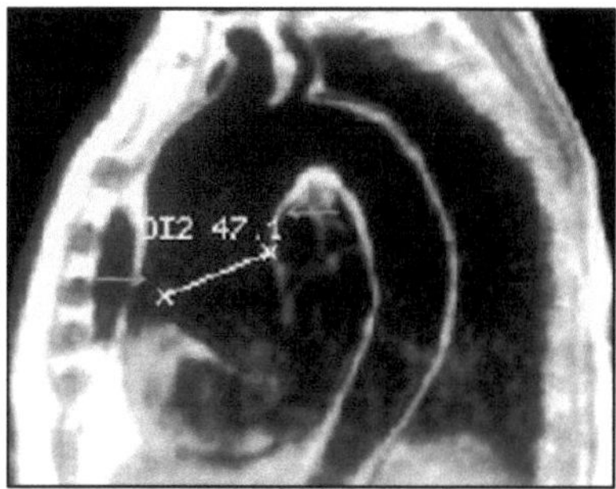

Figure 13: Sagittal reconstruction of a thoracic MRI showing an aneurysm of the ascending aorta in the setting of Horton's disease [53].

7- PET-scan [58]:

PET scanning is a powerful tool for the early diagnosis of large-vessel vasculitis at the initial stage of the disease, even before the appearance of anatomical lesions [59, 60]. It provides a map of damage to the aorta and large- and medium-calibre arterial branches. Its use is recommended by EULAR for diagnosis, alongside MRI [61].

FDG (18-fluoro deoxyglucose) positron emission tomography (PET scan) visualizes the presence of hypermetabolic foci within the arterial wall, showing the presence of arterial hyperfixations.

This examination is therefore of interest in the diagnosis of Takayasu's disease, as it reveals arterial fixations in the context of an unexplained inflammatory syndrome.

Webb et al [62] estimated the sensitivity of FDG PET at 92% and specificity at 100% for the assessment of disease activity.

Various series have studied the performance of PET for the diagnosis of Horton's disease. Its diagnostic sensitivity ranges from 50 to 100%, and its specificity from 95 to 100% in untreated patients [63, 64]. Its sensitivity is increased when inflammation markers are elevated [65]. Blockman et al have reported a specificity of 98% for PET in the diagnosis of Horton's disease, if only FDG uptake in the thoracic aorta is considered [63, 65, 66].

V. Clinical forms :

1- Aneurysm of the subrenal abdominal aorta :

1- 1- Clinical study :

This is the most common location for inflammatory aortic aneurysms.

In 80% of cases, the aneurysm is totally latent, discovered by chance during an ultrasound or abdominal CT scan prompted by urological or digestive pathology, or during routine screening.

In 20% of cases, the aneurysm is revealed by posteriorly radiating epigastric pain, or pain in the lower limbs indicating an embolic complication.

In non-obese patients, clinical examination may reveal a pulsating, expansive abdominal mass in the umbilical region. The sub-renal location of the aneurysm is indicated by the De Bakey sign: if the hand is slipped between the mass and the costal margin, the ectasia is sub-renal.

1- 2- Evolution-Complications :

Ischemic stroke of the lower limbs due to embolism from an intra-aneurysmal thrombus is a classic but rare complication. Aneurysm rupture is the most serious complication. However, the risk of rupture of these inflammatory aneurysms is reduced by the peri-aneurysmal fibrous shell.

Ruptures located in the inferior vena cava or duodenum, or contained by the spine, may be observed more frequently, since the posterior surface of the aneurysm is relatively spared from fibrosis.

Compression and adhesion to neighboring organs, notably the inferior vena cava, duodenum and left renal vein, are specific complications of these inflammatory aneurysms.

The most frequent complications are often urological: in addition to ureteral detour due to retroperitoneal fibrosis, ureteral obstruction is the major evolutionary risk.

2- Aneurysm of the suprarenal abdominal aorta :

2- 1- Clinical study :

Involvement of the supra-renal abdominal aorta is very rare and usually asymptomatic.

When it also affects the mesenteric artery, it can manifest as :

- Abdominal pain.
- Transit disorders such as diarrhea or cessation of feces and gas.

2- 2- Evolution-Complications :

Possible complications include :

- Renovascular hypertension.
- Kidney failure.
- Angina or digestive ischemia in the event of digestive artery involvement
- Adhesion and compression of neighboring components
- The break.

3- Aneurysm of the thoracic aorta :

3- 1- Clinical study :

This is the most common location in Horton's disease.

Evans et al [67] estimated that patients with Horton's disease had a 17.3-fold increased risk of developing a thoracic aortic aneurysm compared with a control population matched for age and cardiovascular risk factors.

Aneurysms of the thoracic aorta are most often asymptomatic, discovered when a complication occurs.

When symptomatic, it can be revealed by : [1]

- Back or chest pain: this is the most common warning sign.
- Dyspnea
- A dry cough
- Aortic arch syndrome, manifested by intermittent claudication of the upper limbs, Raynaud's phenomenon, abolition of a distal pulse or a vascular murmur.

3- 2- Evolution- Complications: [1]

Aneurysms of the thoracic aorta are most often diagnosed as a complication:

- A rupture or dissection
- Aortic insufficiency
- Stroke in the carotid or vertebral territory
- Myocardial infarction

In Horton's disease, aortic dissection occurs on average at 74.5 years of age [68]. It is usually a type II according to the De Bakey classification.

VI. Positive diagnosis :

1- Takayasu disease:

The diagnosis of Takayasu disease is based on a combination of clinical, biological and radiological factors.

Several teams have proposed diagnostic criteria whose practical value remains debatable [69]. These criteria, which are based on arteriography, do not allow diagnosis in the early phase of the disease, before stenoses have become established.

1- 1- Ishikawa diagnostic criteria, modified by Sharma in 1996 [70]:

The first diagnostic criteria were proposed by Ishikawa in 1988 [2].

These criteria were too restrictive, excluding patients aged over 40 at the onset of the disease, and taking into account lesions of the abdominal aorta only if they respect the iliac arteries, whereas the latter are affected in 11 to 30% of cases [70].

In 1996, Sharma et al [70] therefore proposed modifications to the Ishikawa criteria to improve their sensitivity, particularly in patient populations where lesions of the abdominal aorta predominate.

The presence of two major criteria, or one major criterion with two minor criteria, or four minor criteria leads to a diagnosis of Takayasu disease with a sensitivity of 92.5% and a specificity of 95% [70].

- Main criteria :

- Stenosis or occlusion of the middle portion of the left subclavian artery on arteriography

- Stenosis or occlusion of the middle portion of the right subclavian artery on arteriography

- Typical symptoms lasting at least 1 month: claudication, pulse abolition or blood pressure asymmetry, fever, carotid dynia, amaurosis, visual disturbances, syncope, dyspnoea, palpitations.

- Minor criteria :

- Sedimentation rate (VS) greater than 20 mm/h

- Carotidodynia: sensitivity of the carotid arteries to palpation

- Brachial arterial pressure > 140/90 mm Hg or popliteal arterial pressure > 160/90 mm Hg

- Aortic insufficiency or aortic ring dilatation

- Damage to the pulmonary arteries

- Stenosis or occlusion of the middle portion of the left carotid artery on arteriography

- Arteriographic stenosis or occlusion of the distal third of the brachiocephalic arterial trunk

- Arteriographic lesion of the descending thoracic aorta

- Abdominal aortic lesion on arteriography

- Coronary lesion with age < 30 in the absence of dyslipidemia or diabetes

1- 2- Activity criteria :

A global activity criterion has been proposed (NIH criteria), combining inflammatory and ischemic clinical elements, SV, and arteriographic data [71].

NIH (national institute of health) activity criteria for Takayasu disease [71] :

Active disease is defined by the recent onset or worsening of at least 2 of the following criteria:

- Signs of vascular ischemia or inflammation: limb claudication, decreased or absent pulse, vascular murmur or pain, carotid dynia, tension asymmetry in upper or lower limbs.

- Systemic signs: fever, arthralgias, myalgias (in the absence of any other identifiable cause)

- Increased sedimentation rate.

- Typical arteriographic abnormalities.

In addition to these classic criteria of disease activity, we can add the progressive or non-progressive nature of vascular thickenings identified on arterial Doppler ultrasound, angiography-CT or angiography-MRI, and vascular wall hyperfixations found on PET scans [6].

The criteria for remission are :

- Complete resolution or stabilization of all clinical signs

- Stable vascular lesions

2- Behçet's disease :

Diagnosis of this vasculitis is based on clinical criteria, essentially those defined by the International Study Group for Behçet's Disease [3]. These criteria have a sensitivity of 91% and a specificity of 96%.

Note that they are applicable only in the absence of other clinical explanations.

Behçet's disease: international criteria 1990 [4] :

- Recurrent oral aphthosis

- 3 types: major, minor, herpetiform

- 3 flare-ups/year

- observed by a physician or by the patient

Plus at least 2 of the following criteria:

- Recurrent genital ulceration or scarring observed by a physician or by the patient.

- Eye damage :

    Anterior uveitis, posterior uveitis, slit lamp hyalitis

    Retinal vasculitis observed by an ophthalmologist

- Skin lesions :

    Erythema nodosum, pseudofolliculitis, papulopustular lesions

    Acne nodules observed by a physician outside adolescence or corticosteroid treatment

- Positive skin test read by a physician after 24 to 48 hours.

3- Horton's disease :

Diagnostic criteria for Horton's disease were established in 1990 by *The* American College *Of* Rheumatology [72].

Diagnostic criteria for giant cell arteritis 1990 [72] :

- Age > 50

- Recent headaches

- Sensitivity to palpation of the temporal artery and/or decrease in temporal pulse

- Sedimentation rate > 50 mm/h.

- A temporal artery biopsy showing vasculitis, arterial necrosis, lymphocytic infiltrate or giant cell granuloma.

The combination of 3 of these 5 criteria establishes the diagnosis with a sensitivity of 95.3% and a specificity of 90.7%.

VII. Differential diagnosis :

Certain differential diagnoses need to be considered in the presence of inflammatory aortitis, as their management is quite different. First and foremost, an infectious cause of aortitis must be ruled out, as its rapid progression and short-term prognosis make it a therapeutic emergency. Secondly, PRF, IG4-associated disease, Erdheim-Chester disease and atheromatous inflammatory aneurysms are other diagnoses to be considered, in order to best adapt the management of these patients.

VIII. Processing :

1- Medical treatment :

The treatment of inflammatory aortitis is based on two therapeutic approaches: medical treatment based on corticosteroid therapy and immunosuppressants, and surgical or endovascular treatment of the aortic lesion.

Medical treatment should be initiated as soon as possible under close clinical supervision to avoid the risk of fatal rupture.

Non-steroidal anti-inflammatory drugs have a clear effect on the articular manifestations of Behçet's disease.

Colchicine is an immunomodulator used at a dosage of 1 to 2 mg/d. A positive response is obtained in 60-70% of cases, essentially for mucocutaneous and articular manifestations. Colchicine also has a role in preventing relapses [73].

Corticosteroid therapy is not justified in cases of isolated mucocutaneous or joint involvement. It is indicated in forms with ocular and neurological involvement. Preoperative administration of high-dose corticosteroids reduces inflammation and pre-aortic fibrosis, and simplifies the surgical procedure.

Anti-coagulants are proposed in cases of arterial and deep-vein thrombosis. They are also prescribed in preventive doses after prosthetic bypass surgery.

Immunosuppressive treatment is reserved for major forms of the disease threatening vital and/or functional prognosis.

According to EULAR recommendations [74], vascular involvement justifies the systematic use of immunosuppressants.

In arterial disease, the prognosis is vital. First-line treatment with cyclophosphamide (Endoxan*) or azathiopirine (Imurel*) seems imperative [75]. Several experts have highlighted the benefits of combining corticosteroids, immunosuppressants and anticoagulants to prevent post-operative occlusive and aneurysmal recurrence, even after endovascular treatment [76].

The treatment of Takayasu disease is based on medical therapy to treat the inflammatory component of the disease, as well as the consequences of the pathology, such as hypertension, and revascularization by angioplasty or surgery [77].

The dose of corticosteroids should then be adapted to the evolution of the inflammatory syndrome and clinical symptoms [6].

Damage to the abdominal aorta associated with retroperitoneal fibrosis and ureteral obstruction requires prolonged corticosteroid therapy, combined with double-J ureteral catheterization, or in the event of failure and/or complete obstruction, percutaneous nephrostomy [78].

Second-line treatment is empirically based on methotrexate (20-25 mg/kg per week), or more recently azathioprine (2 mg/kg per day) [79, 80]. Mycophenolate mofetil and anti-TNF (Tumor Necrosis Factor) may be therapeutic alternatives in forms resistant to corticosteroid treatment and conventional immunosuppressants [81].

Hypertension should be managed in the conventional way, bearing in mind the frequency of renal artery stenosis [5]. Medical treatment of hypertension mainly involves beta-blockers, calcium channel blockers, renin-angiotensin system enzyme inhibitors and diuretics [25].

2- Surgical treatment :

Surgical aortitis is often operated on in the sequelae stage, after inflammatory disease has caused irreversible damage to the aortic wall.

One of the challenges of this type of prosthetic surgery is the risk of sepsis. Indeed, patients treated with immunosuppressive drugs are exposed to the risk of infectious contamination of their vascular prosthesis, which can be extremely serious.

In urgent cases (fissure syndrome, acute dissection, very large aneurysms, acute ischemia of the digestive tract, kidneys or lower limbs), the vital risk takes precedence over the infectious risk, and surgery must be performed despite a higher dose of immunosuppressive therapy.

2- 1- Preoperative assessment :

- **Respiratory status:** Respiratory complications are a major cause of post-operative morbidity, and warrant systematic pre-operative assessment.

The preoperative work-up should take into account the patient's previous pneumological history, the existence of smoking intoxication, and the clinical repercussions of any respiratory insufficiency. This clinical workup is complemented by a chest X-ray, and possibly a pulmonary function test and arterial blood gas.

- **Search for associated aneurysms :** The association of one or more arterial aneurysms is quite frequent, especially in Behçet's disease, which makes it necessary to systematically search for them preoperatively.

Associated thoracic aneurysms should be detected by chest X-ray and CT scan of the thoracic aorta in conjunction with the abdominal aorta. Femoral and popliteal aneurysms are palpable on clinical examination.

- **Hypertension and renal function:** Hypertension plays a decisive role in the genesis and growth of aneurysms. Similarly, preoperative renal function tests are warranted to detect renal insufficiency, which may require special precautions.

- **Cardiac status:** Cardiac status should be assessed by looking for a history of myocardial infarction, angina pain, electrocardiogram analysis, cardiac ultrasound, and possibly coronary angiography.

2- 2- Gestures performed :

Some authors recommend the use of homografts in the surgical treatment of inflammatory aneurysms [82].

- **Sub-renal abdominal aortic aneurysm:** transperitoneal vertical midline laparotomy allows wide access to the entire abdominal cavity, and offers the possibility of supra-renal clamping [78].

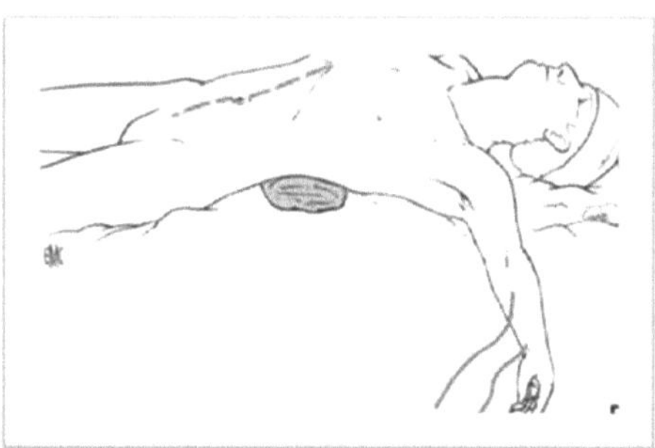

Figure 14: Vertical median laparotomy [78].

Use of the transverse approach reduces the frequency of ventrations and respiratory complications.

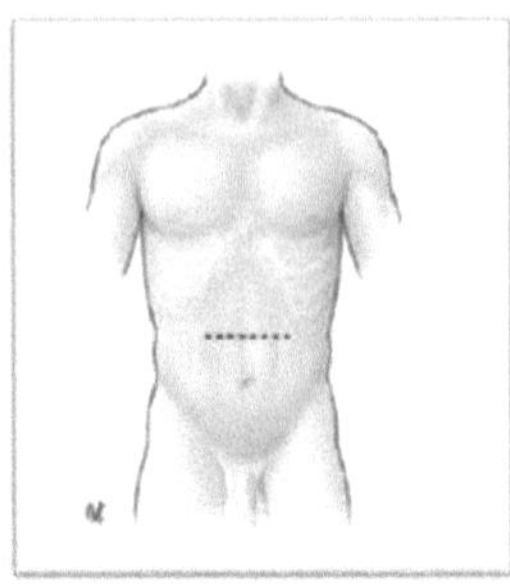

Figure 15: Transverse laparotomy respecting the broad abdominal muscles [83].

The posterior or retroperitoneal approach is an excellent choice for inflammatory aneurysms, as it avoids dissection of neighbouring organs [84]. In addition, it has better respiratory tolerance.

After vertical midline laparotomy, the duodenum and small intestines are retracted. Control of the aorta upstream of the aneurysm is performed after incision of the peritoneum.

These aneurysms are also characterized by the presence of a retroperitoneal fibrous shell, located on the anterior and lateral surfaces of the aorta, and creating very tight adhesions with neighboring organs, in particular the duodenum, ureters, inferior vena cava and left renal vein. Fibrosis can lead to unilateral or bilateral ureteral obstruction, resulting in upstream pyelo-caliceal dilatation. This fibrosis makes aortic dissection and control difficult [85].

Any attempt to dissect the aneurysm may result in damage to neighboring organs, notably the duodenum.

The safest technique is to check the supra-aneurysmal aorta in a healthy supra-renal or celiac zone. Clamping of the iliac arteries is best performed endovascularly, using an occlusive probe to avoid venous or ureteral injury. When the inferior mesenteric artery is permeable, it is checked as close as possible to its ostium [78].

After general heparinization and clamping of the aorta and iliac arteries, the aneurysmal pocket is opened longitudinally, the parietal thrombus is evacuated, and aortic continuity is restored by fitting a Dacron or PTFE prosthesis.

In the case of aneurysms strictly localized to the sub-renal aorta, aorto-aortic tubing is used to restore aortic continuity. If, on the other hand, the aneurysm continues into the iliac arteries, an aorto-iliac prosthesis is inserted.

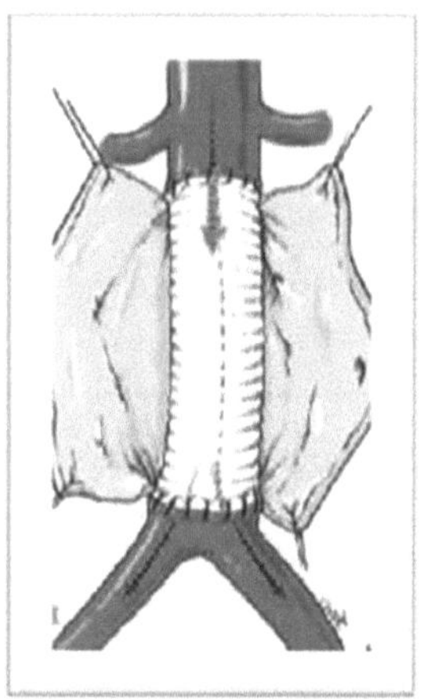

Figure 16: Aorto-aortic prosthesis in place [78].

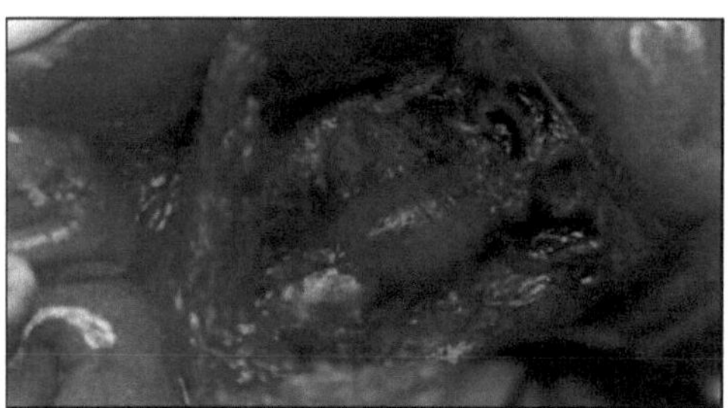

Figure 17: Intraoperative view showing placement of an aorto-aortic prosthesis after resection of the aneurysm in a patient with Behçet's disease.

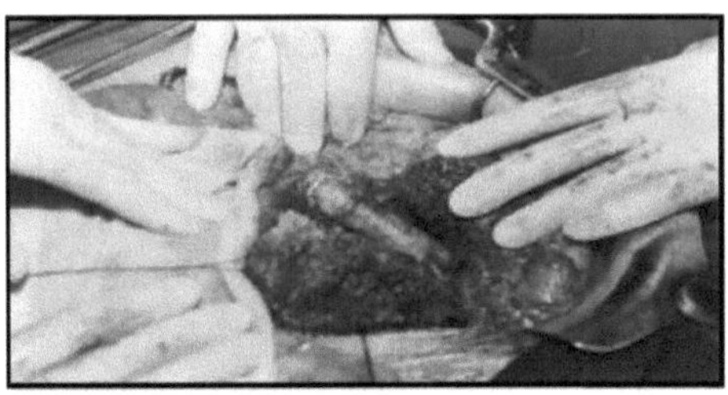

Figure 18: Intraoperative view showing placement of a bifurcated prosthesis after resection of the aneurysm.

If the inferior mesenteric artery is permeable, it must be re-implanted onto the prosthesis. The procedure is completed by closing the aneurysmal pocket around the prosthesis to prevent infection of the prosthesis from contact with the duodenum.

The anastomoses between the prosthesis and the aorta must be protected to avoid the development of a false anastomotic aneurysm.

Aortic aneurysms in Behçet's disease pose particular problems. These are often saccular aneurysms, for which resection with patch enlargement may be indicated [86].

This is a simple technique used by some authors to treat false saccular aneurysms. It involves limited dissection of the aneurysm, clamping of the aorta upstream and downstream, and opening of the sac. The neck is closed with a Dacron patch.

Obstruction of the urinary tract by fibrosis in abdominal aortic aneurysms, which is characteristic of inflammatory aneurysms, justifies the use of an endoscopic drainage device in all cases, regardless of the surgical management of the aneurysm.

Aortic clamping causes hemodynamic disturbances, the extent of which depends on the level of clamping, the size of the downstream bed and the pre-operative myocardial state.

Prevention of post-operative renal failure is ensured by maintaining hemodynamic stability during the operation. Correct blood volume must be maintained by compensating for insensible losses caused by the externalization of the small intestines, and for blood losses using filling solutions and blood products.

- **Aneurysms of the ascending aorta :** Aneurysms of the ascending aorta are common in Horton's disease. In non-emergency situations, it is advisable to operate on a patient in clinical and biological remission, in order to limit the risk of suture loosening when operating on an inflamed aorta.

At this level, three types of lesions are likely to be associated:

- Aortic insufficiency due to direct damage or dilatation of the aortic annulus
- Occlusive lesions of the coronary arteries
- Ascending aortic aneurysm
- Replacement of the ascending aorta may be proposed in cases of coronary artery bypass surgery for occlusive lesions of the coronary arteries, or in cases where the diameter of the ascending aorta exceeds 50 mm. However, the sometimes thickened and fibrous nature of the ascending aorta may prevent the implantation of a saphenous bypass under good conditions. Furthermore, the frequent involvement of the

supra-aortic trunks, and in particular the subclavian arteries, in Takayasu's disease contraindicates the use of mammary arteries in this case [87].

In the case of a large aortic leak associated with an aneurysm of the ascending aorta, it must be corrected surgically [25]. In this case, a Bentall operation is indicated.

- **Aneurysm of the aortic arch:** The aortic arch poses greater technical and technological difficulties, due to its angulations, the origin of the supra-aortic trunks and the proximity of the aortic valve.

The surgical approach to the aortic arch can be difficult, given the anatomical features outlined above. Sternotomy is the approach of choice, as it is simple and minimally traumatic, and offers excellent exposure for anterior and horizontal arch aneurysms. It enables endo-aneurysmal replacement of the saphenofemoral junction.

Lesions that do not extend beyond the isthmus can be treated by sternotomy. Lesions of the crossover beginning after the left primary carotid artery and lesions of the descending thoracic aorta require left posterolateral thoracotomy.

More extensive lesions involving the ascending aorta, the crossover and extending into the descending thoracic aorta represent a major surgical challenge [88].

- **Aneurysms of the descending thoracic and thoracoabdominal aorta**: Aortic aneurysms in Takayasu disease usually occur in the thoracoabdominal aorta [89]. The incidence of thoracoabdominal aneurysms is around 10% [90, 91].

Aortic aneurysms in Takayasu disease are frequently associated with stenoses of the digestive tract, which can also contribute to the indication for aortic replacement despite a diameter of less than 60 mm.

In the series by Kieffer et al [90], 58% of the 33 patients who underwent thoracoabdominal aortic replacement had required visceral revascularization for stenotic lesions.

- **Ruptured aneurysms:** Inflammatory aneurysms can lead to severe complications such as rupture [92]. In addition to increased pain, they are characterized by hemodynamic instability and deglobulation.

They require vascular filling and emergency intervention.

Umehara et al [92] reported a case of ruptured aneurysm of the thoracoabdominal aorta associated with Behçet's disease, treated by placement of a cryopreserved homograft, under thoraco-phreno-lumbotomy and femoral-femoral extracorporeal circulation.

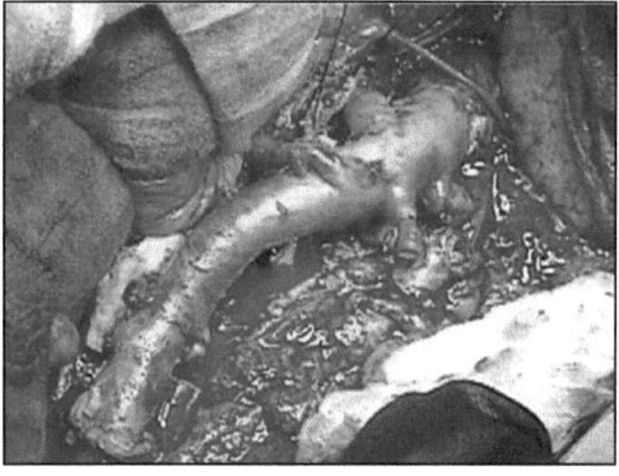

Figure 19: Intraoperative photograph showing the aortic homograft with its main branches [92].

3- Endovascular treatment :

Endovascular treatment of aneurysms by interposition of covered stents enables exclusion of the aneurysm sac and restoration of arterial continuity, without direct approach to the aneurysm, and without the morbidity associated with incisions and surgical detachments. It is a good alternative given the surgical difficulties associated with inflammatory adhesions, the frequency of recurrences, and false anastomotic aneurysms.

However, the implementation of this technique comes up against several types of difficulties resulting from the morphology of the aneurysm and linked to the very principles of the technique:

- Stenting requires a surgical approach to the Scarpas, due to the size of the introducers.

- The permeability of the lumbar arteries and/or inferior mesenteric artery may make it difficult to achieve complete thrombosis of the abdominal aortic aneurysm pocket around the stent graft.

- Stenting requires a proximal collar of around 20 mm to ensure solid fixation of the stent.

- In the absence of a distal aortic neck, a bifurcated stent graft must be used in abdominal aortic aneurysms.

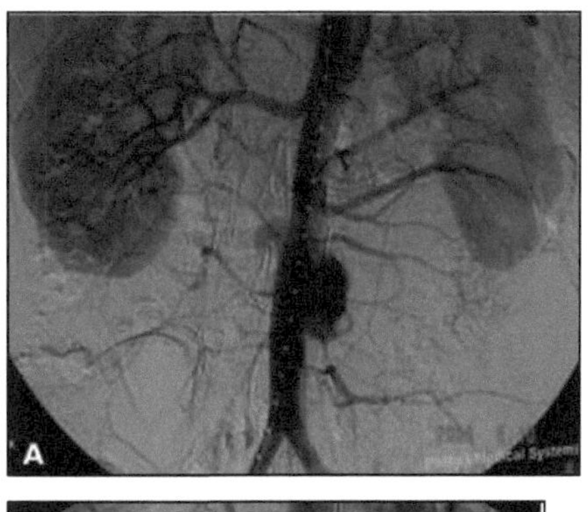

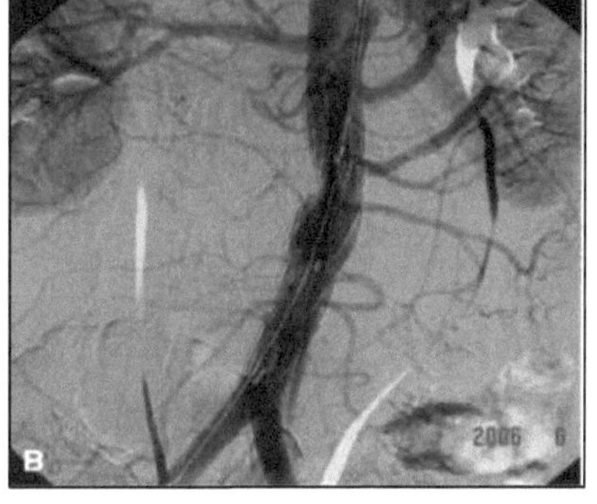

Figure 20: A: False aneurysm of the subrenal aorta.

B: exclusion of false aneurysm by a covered stent graft [93].

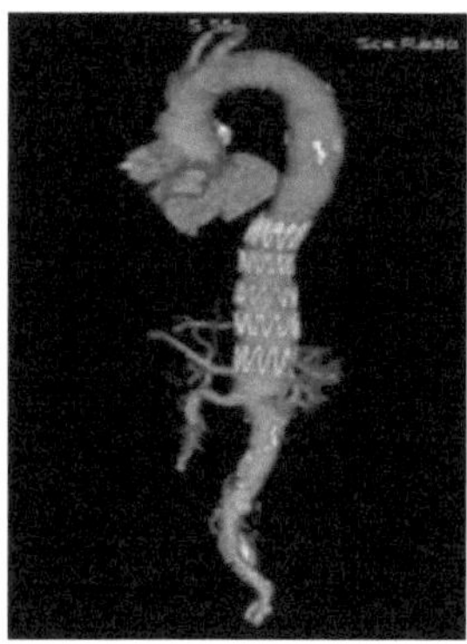

Figure 21: False inflammatory aneurysm of the supra-celiac aorta treated with tubular covered stent grafting, with total collapse of the aneurysmal lesion.

Unlike the thoracoabdominal aorta, where fenestrated and branched prostheses allow perfusion of the major collateral branches of the aorta from the tubular aortic stent graft, the complexity of the anatomy of the arch limits a pure endovascular solution to a few clinical cases at present [94]. It is therefore essential to preserve the supra-aortic trunks by rerouting them: stents specially designed for the thoracic aorta, with prior rerouting of the supra-aortic trunks by cervical approach or sternotomy, are used for pathology of the distal horizontal aorta [88].

4- Indications [87]:

The management of inflammatory aneurysms follows the same guidelines as those for degenerative aneurysms. Indications for surgery must take into account the characteristics of the aneurysm: size, progression and functional symptomatology, so as to propose surgery to prevent rupture.

In addition to the anatomical-clinical indications for surgical treatment, the indications selected must take into account the patient's general condition, so as to propose a procedure with a reasonable operative risk.

A diameter greater than 50 mm in the ascending aorta, 60 mm in the descending thoracic aorta, and 50 mm in the abdominal aorta justifies prosthetic grafting.

In the case of aneurysms of the abdominal sub-renal aorta, the surgical indication is formal when :

- A symptomatic aneurysm of any size

- A ruptured or rupturing aneurysm

- An asymptomatic aortic aneurysm whose size exceeds 50 mm in diameter, given the high risk of rupture.

Small, painless false aneurysms with no signs of rupture can be monitored and treated medically [95].

Conventional surgical treatment is most often used for aneurysms associated with aortitis, although more recently, cases of endovascular treatment have been reported with a satisfactory early success rate.

Endovascular treatment has the advantage of avoiding the manipulation of highly inflammatory tissues, but no comparative studies have been carried out, and not uncommon cases of false aneurysms occurring opposite proximal stents have been reported.

Cracked or ruptured aneurysms are an indication for emergency surgery.

5- Therapeutic results :

5- 1- Early results :

The results of surgery for inflammatory aneurysms of the sub-renal abdominal aorta are good, as the procedure is generally performed in young, non-tart subjects.

In abdominal aortic surgery, dissection is made more difficult by inflammatory phenomena, resulting in an increased risk of hemorrhage and intraoperative damage to the duodenum, vena cava and ureters [96].

Biological markers of inflammation are generally elevated after conventional surgery [96].

Possible post-operative complications are [97]:

- Haemorrhage due to early release of sutures on fragile, inflammatory arteries.

- Colonic ischemia: this is a serious complication of abdominal aortic aneurysm surgery, characterized by a combination of diarrhea, left iliac fossa pain and rectorrhagia, associated with a febrile state [78]. It usually occurs from 36ème hours post-operatively, but may occur later.

Diagnosis is based on colonoscopy. Treatment is based on surgical removal of the colon.

- Renal failure: favored by preoperative occlusive damage to the renal arteries, suprarenal aortic clamping, and intraoperative hemodynamic variations.

- Sexual complications such as retrograde ejaculation due to sectioning of the presacral nerves.

- Neurological complications such as spinal cord ischemia due to abnormal birth of Adamkiewicz's artery.

- Prosthesis thrombosis: treatment is surgical thrombectomy.

- Prosthesis infections: the risks are heightened by the fact that this is a difficult surgery in a special situation (patients on corticosteroids). This is a rare and serious complication, with a high morbidity and mortality rate.

- A particular complication of ASD surgery, due to the often severe and diffuse ASD involvement, is postoperative reperfusion syndrome, sometimes responsible for intracerebral hemorrhage [98]. For this reason, strict intra- and post-operative blood pressure control is recommended in such cases. This requires prior treatment of any renal-vascular hypertension. Because of the high recurrence rate, particularly at sites of arterial trauma, the risk of recurrence at the anastomosis site is greater than in other aortic diseases. Aneurysmorrhaphies with patch closure are associated with a high recurrence rate, ranging from 17% [95] to 66% [99], and should be preferred to prosthetic grafts.

The mortality rate after endovascular treatment is lower than that after open surgery [96]. Indeed, the mortality rate after endovascular treatment of inflammatory aneurysms of the abdominal aorta is in the order of 0-2.4% in the most recent series [96].

Possible intraoperative complications of endovascular treatment of aortic aneurysms and false aneurysms are :

- Complications at the puncture site: Possible complications include hematoma and false aneurysm.

- Stent maldeployment: Deployment may be supplemented by ballooning.

- Stent loosening

- Arterial rupture: requires surgical repair or placement of a covered stent.

Endovascular treatment of aortic aneurysms may be associated with an inflammatory reaction known as "post-implantation syndrome", characterized by abdominal and lumbar pain associated with hyperthermia above 38° C, as well as a biological inflammatory syndrome in the days following stent implantation, irrespective of pre-existing inflammation [96].

The frequency of post-implantation syndrome varies from 14 to 60% of cases [97]. The type of stent also seems to play a role in the intensity and frequency of this syndrome, with polyester (Dacron) appearing to be associated with a greater inflammatory reaction than polytetrafluoroethylene (PTFE) [98].

Biological markers of inflammation are generally elevated after endovascular treatment, irrespective of the occurrence of a post-implantation syndrome. CRP, for example, generally rises until the 3rd postoperative day and then falls within a month of stent implantation [99]. SV, white blood cells and platelets increase progressively up to day 7 after endovascular treatment, CRP and interleukin 6 earlier, after 48 and 24 hours respectively.

The procalcitonin assay appears to be a more specific marker of infection [100].

Post-implantation syndrome has long led to the belief that endovascular management of inflammatory aortic aneurysms risks exacerbating inflammatory phenomena, with a corollary worsening of fibrosing phenomena. However, as early as the 2000s, some authors reported a few cases of patients treated with stents for inflammatory aortic aneurysms without any notable complications during follow-up [101].

Other early complications after endovascular treatment of aortic aneurysms are :

- **Primary endoleaks:** These are defined by the existence of persistent or recurrent blood flow between the stent-graft and the arterial wall.

Type 1 endoleaks, located in the stent anchoring zones, require stent extension if the leak is large, or surgical conversion if the endovascular procedure is not possible.

Type 2 endoleaks, arising from an arterial branch covered by the stent, in this case the internal iliac artery, are the most common.

Type 3 and 4 endoleaks are extremely rare.

Type 3 endoleaks are linked to a leak at the junction of two parts, or to dislocation of the components of a modular stent. Type 4 endoleaks are linked to microleaks due to porosity at the sutures between the metal components making up the stent framework. Moderate endoleaks detected on CT should be monitored regularly.

- **Stent migration:** Migration of a stent requires surgical removal.

Late complications include :

- **False anastomotic aneurysms:** whatever treatment is adopted, it does not rule out the occurrence of progressive complications such as a new aneurysmal localization or a false anastomotic aneurysm, the rate of which is particularly high in inflammatory aortic disease.

False anastomotic aneurysms are dilatations consisting of thrombus, prosthesis, native arterial wall and inflammatory tissue.

Aneurysmorrhaphy with patch closure is associated with a higher recurrence rate than flattening with prosthetic grafting, ranging from 17% [95] to 66% [99], and should be preferred to prosthetic grafting.

In the study by Tuzun et al [102], the risk of recurrence or appearance of a new aneurysm was 22% under immunosuppressive treatment in cases of arterial involvement, regardless of location. For specific cases of aortic involvement, the recurrence rate ranged from 14% to 45%.

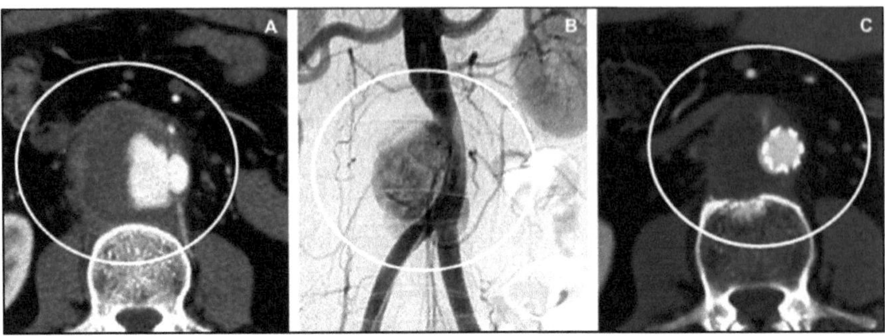

Figure 22: Angioscan showing false aneurysm on enlargement patch [103].

Prosthetic-digestive fistulas are a rare but severe complication after aortic reconstruction surgery. They are secondary to the rupture of anastomotic pseudoaneurysms of the prosthetic grafts. Their frequency is between 0.4% and 4% [104].

They manifest themselves as upper digestive haemorrhage, sometimes massive, occurring several months to several years after the operation [104]. Diagnosis is based on digestive endoscopy.

Removal of the prosthesis and digestive resection are necessary. They are often combined with extra-anatomical revascularization.

Iscan et al [105] reported a case of prosthetic duodenal fistula complicating surgery for a pseudoaneurysm of the abdominal aorta due to Behçet's disease, treated by duodenal resection with anatomical revascularization via a rifampicin-impregnated aorto-aortic tube and omentoplasty.

The risk of bypass restenosis or thrombosis occurs in 8% to 31% of cases after 3 to 6 years of follow-up [106].

In the study by Paravastu et al [107], the benefit in terms of one-year mortality was even greater after endovascular surgery than after conventional surgery: (2% versus 14% and p = 0.02) in the treatment of inflammatory aneurysms of the abdominal aorta.

In a meta-analysis by Puchner et al [108], the evolution of periaortic fibrosis following endovascular treatment was as follows: complete regression in 51.2% of cases, no change in 41.8% and progression in 7%.

In another meta-analysis, fibrosis regressed more often and more completely after open surgery than after endovascular surgery: regression observed in 86% of cases after open surgery versus 60% after endovascular treatment [109].

In patients with pre-operative hydronephrosis, open surgery appears to be more beneficial in terms of urological outcome. In the study by Paravastu et al [107], hydronephrosis regressed in 69% of cases after conventional surgical treatment versus 38% of cases after endovascular treatment (p = 0.01).

All in all, postoperative complications in the treatment of inflammatory aortic disease remain serious and fatal. A review of the literature shows that endovascular treatment may reduce peri-operative mortality, but has failed to reduce medium- or short-term complications.

Aortic involvement in inflammatory diseases is therefore serious. Even when treated, it can be life-threatening due to fatal complications. Screening for such damage in patients with systemic disease, and regular radiological follow-up of treated patients, are essential for early detection and management of complications.

IX. Conclusion:

Inflammatory aortitis is dominated by Takayasu's disease, Horton's disease and Behçet's disease.

Takayasu's disease is an inflammatory arteritis of the large vessels, primarily affecting the aorta and its main branches. It affects young people and manifests itself mainly as multiple arterial stenoses.

Behçet's disease is a systemic vasculitis of as yet obscure etiology, evolving in successive attacks and affecting vessels of all calibers. It is associated with involvement of large-caliber vessels, individualized within a framework known as angio-Behçet and subdivided into venous involvement, which is very frequent, and arterial involvement, which is less frequent.

Horton's disease affects the elderly, and is mainly responsible for aortic aneurysms, with the risk of rupture a major factor in its severity.

Diagnosis of inflammatory aortitis is based on imaging. At present, echo-Doppler, angio-CT and MRI are reliable and rapid methods for assessing vessel lumina and walls.

Clinical expression varies according to the nature of the lesion, its location and associated lesions:

- Aneurysms of the thoracic aorta are usually asymptomatic, discovered when a complication occurs. When they are symptomatic, they may be revealed by chest pain (the most frequent warning sign), dyspnea, dry cough, aortic arch syndrome, neurological signs or coronary syndrome.

- Involvement of the supra-renal abdominal aorta is often asymptomatic. When it also affects the mesenteric artery, it may manifest as abdominal pain or transit disorders. It may be revealed by hypertension or renal failure, often secondary to renal artery stenosis.

- Aneurysms of the abdominal sub-renal aorta are asymptomatic in 80% of cases. When symptomatic, it may present as posteriorly radiating epigastric pain or lower limb pain, reflecting an embolic complication.

Recent advances in the diagnosis of aortic disease have involved the use of non-invasive imaging techniques to diagnose aortic disease, assess the extent of lesions and monitor progress under treatment.

Surgical treatment of inflammatory aortic disease represents a challenge for the vascular surgeon, due to the intraoperative difficulties involved, the frequency of postoperative complications and the possibility of new aneurysm formation, hence the need to establish the right surgical indications and always combine them with effective medical treatment.

Surgery is required for any symptomatic abdominal aortic aneurysm, regardless of size, for any ruptured or cracked aneurysm, or for any asymptomatic aortic aneurysm with a diameter in excess of 50 mm, given the high risk of rupture. For thoracic aortic aneurysms, a diameter greater than 50 mm in the ascending aorta, 60 mm in the descending thoracic aorta, or a complicated aneurysm, justifies prosthetic grafting.

Endovascular techniques and equipment have progressed over the last 10 years, and the number of patients benefiting from these techniques continues to grow. Endovascular treatment Endovascular treatment is a good alternative, given the surgical difficulties associated with inflammatory adhesions, the frequency of recurrences, and the risk of false anastomotic aneurysms.

Endoluminal treatment of aneurysms by interposition of covered stents enables exclusion of the aneurysm sac and restoration of arterial continuity, without direct approach to the aneurysm, and without the morbidity associated with incisions and surgical detachments.

However, post-operative complications are frequent, dominated by graft thrombosis, false anastomotic aneurysms and prosthetic-digestive fistulas. The mortality rate after endovascular treatment is lower than after open surgery.

Possible intraoperative complications of endovascular treatment of aortic aneurysms include hematomas, false aneurysms at the puncture site, stent graft maldeployment, stent graft loosening and arterial rupture.

Endovascular treatment of aortic aneurysms may also be associated with an inflammatory reaction known as "post-implantation syndrome", characterized by abdominal and lumbar pain associated with hyperthermia above 38°C, and a biological inflammatory syndrome in the days following stent implantation, irrespective of pre-existing inflammation.

Bibliography :

[1] Launay D, Hachulla E. Les aortites inflammatoires. Presse Med 2004; 33: 1334-40.

[2] Ishikawa K. Diagnostic approach and proposed criteria for the clinical diagnosis of Takayasu's arteriopathy. J Am Coll Cardiol 1988; 12: 964-72.

[3] International Study Group For Behçet's Disease. Criteria for the diagnosis of Behçet's disease. Lancet 1990 :335 : 1078-80.

[4] Raglianti V, Rossi GM, Vaglio A. Idiopathic retroperitoneal fibrosis: an update for nephrologists. Nephrol Dial Transpl 2020; 36: 1773-81

[5] Arnaud L, Haroche J, Piette J.C, Amoura Z. Takayasu's arteritis: an update on a mono-centric series of 82 patients. La Revue de médecine interne 2010 ; 31 :208-215.

[6] Thomas Quéméneur, Éric Hachulla, Marc Lambert, Maryse Perez-Cousin, Viviane Queyrel, David Launay, Sandrine Morell-Dubois, Pierre-Yves Hatron. Takayasu disease. Presse Med 2006; 35: 847-56.

[7] Wechsler B, Dul T, Kieffer E. Cardiovascular manifestations of Behçet's disease. Ann MedInterne1999; 150: 542-54.

[8] Wechsler B, Asli B, Le Thi Houng Du et al. Aortic involvement and Behçet's disease. JMV 2008; 12: 084.

[9] Cormier JM, Cormier F, Laridon D, Vuong PN. Horton's disease and aortic aneurysm: coincidence or association? Five observations. J Mal Vasc 2000; 25: 92-7.

[10] Sharma S, Rajani M, Talwar KK. Angiographic morphology in nonspecific aortoarteritis (Takayasu's arteritis): a study of 126 patients from north India. Cardiovasc Intervent Radiol 1992;15: 160-5.

[11] Park MC, Lee SW, Park YB, Chung NS, Lee SK. Clinical characteristics and outcomes of Takayasu's arteritis: analysis of 108 patients using standardized criteria for diagnosis, activity assessment, and angiographic classification. Scand J Rheumatol 2005; 34: 284-92.

[12] Mwipatayi BP, Jeffery PC, BeningfieldSJ, Matley PJ, Naidoo NG, Kalla AA, et al. Takayasu arteritis: clinical features and management: report of272 cases. ANZ J Surg 2005; 75: 110-7.

[13] Lupi-Herrera E, Sanchez-Torres G, Marcushamer J, Mispireta J, HorwitzS, Vela JE. Takayasu's arteritis. Clinical study of 107 cases. Am Heart J 1977; 93: 94-103.

[14] Fiessinger JN, Paul JF.Aortites. Rev Prat 2002; 52: 1094-9.

[15] Vanoli M, Daina E, Salvarani C, Sabbadini MG, Rossi C, Bacchiani G, et al. Takayasu's arteritis: a study of 104 Italian patients. Arthritis Rheum 2005; 53: 100-7.

[16] Cakar N, Yalcinkaya F, Duzova A, Caliskan S, Sirin A, Oner A, et al. Takayasu arteritis in children. J Rheumatol 2008; 35: 913-9.

[17] Arend WP, Michel BA, Bloch DA, Hunder GG, Calabrese LH, Edworthy SM, et al. The American College of Rheumatology 1990 criteriafor the classification of Takayasu arteritis. Arthritis Rheum 1990; 33: 1129-34.

[18] Hall S, Barr W, Lie JT, Stanson AW, Kazmier FJ, Hunder GG. Takayasu arteritis. A study of 32 North American patients. Medicine (Baltimore). 1985; 64:89-99.

[19] Ko GY, Byun JY, Choi BG, Cho SH. The vascular manifestations of Behçet's disease: angiographic andCT findings. Br J Radiol 2000; 73: 1270-4.

[20] Besbas N, Ozyurek E, Balkanci F et al. Behçet's disease with severe arterial involvement in a child. Clin Rheumatol 2002, 21(2): 176-179.

[21] Marie Bossert, Clément Prati, Jean-Charles Balblanc, Anne Lohse, Daniel Wendling. Aortic involvement in Horton's disease: current aspects. Société française de rhumatologie. Elsevier Masson SAS. 2010.08.004.

[22] Le Tourneau T, Millaire A, Asseman P, De Groote P, Théry C, Ducloux G. Horton's aortitis. Ann Med Interne 1996; 147: 361-8.

[23] Evans JM, O'Fallon WM, Hunder GG. Increased incidence of aortic aneurysm and dissection in giant cell (temporal) arteritis. A population based study. Ann Intern Med 1995; 122: 502-7.

[24] Wissem Ellouze. Digestive artery revascularization, indications, techniques and results. A propos de 17 cas. 2014. Thesis of medicine. Faculté de médecine de Sfax.

[25] Tristan Mirault, Joseph Emmerich. Takayasu disease. How to manage it? Presse Med. 2012; 41: 975-985.

[26] Wechsler B, Le Thi Huong DU. Behçet's disease. La revue du praticien (Paris) 1996, 46 p 1316-22.

[27] Lina Benabdellaoui Arterial involvement in Behçet's disease. Thèse de médecine. Faculté de médecine de Sfax 2010.

[28] Sakane T, Takeno M, Inaba G. Behçet's disease. N Engl J Med 1999; 341(17): 1284 -91.

[29] Charles Masson. Therapeutic approach to giant cell vasculitis (Horton's disease). Société française de rhumatologie. Elsevier Masson SAS. 2011.

[30] Marie I, Proux A, Duhaut P, Primard E, Lahaxe L, Girszyn N et al. Long-term follow-up of aortic involvement in giant cell arteritis: a series of 48 patients. Medicine 2009; 88(3): 182-92.

[31] Raninen RO, Pamilo MS, Leirisalo-Repo KT, Hekali PE. Graft patency evaluation with colour Doppler ultrasonography after bypass surgery in Takayasu's arteritis: a direct colour-flow lumen imaging method. Eur J 1998; 16: 525-9.

[32] Lefebvre C, Rance A, Paul JF et al. The role of B-mode ultrasonography and electron beam computed tomography in evaluation of Takayasu's arteritis: a study of 43 patients. Semin Arthritis Rheum 2000; 30: 25-32.

[33] Aluquin P, Albano SA, Chan F, Sandborg C, Pitlick PT. Magnetic resonance imaging in the diagnosis and follow-up of Takayasu's arteritis in children. Ann Rheum Dis 2002; 61: 526-9.

[34] Hoffman GS, Ahmed AE. Surrogate markers of disease activity in patients with takayasu arteritis. A preliminary report from the international networkfor the study of the systemic vasculitides (inssys). Int J Cardiol 1998; 66 (Suppl. 1): S191-4.

[35] Arnaud L, Haroche J, Gambotti L, Limal N, Cacoub P, Le-Thi-Huong Boutin D, et al. Takayasu disease: monocentric retrospective study of 82 cases. Rev Med Interne 2006; 27(Suppl. 3): S327-8.

[36] Hoffman GS. Takayasu arteritis: lessons from the American National Institutes of Health experience. Int J Cardiol 1996;(Suppl. 54): S99-102.

[37] Hamza M, Ayed K, Zribi A. Maladie de Behçet. Les manifestations systémiques ; Khan MF, Peltier AP, Ed Flammarion 1991, P 917-947.

[38] Hamzaoui K, Kesraoui A. Immunology of Behçet's disease. Tunisie Med 1990, 68 n° 2, 101-104.

[39] Evans JM, Hunder GG. The implications of recognizing large-vessel involvement in elderly patients with giant cell arteritis. Curr Opin Rheumatol 1997; 9: 37-40.

[40] Sun Y, Yip PK, Jeng JS, Hwang BS, Lin WH. Ultrasonographic study and long-term follow-up of Takayasu's arteritis. Stroke 1996; 27: 2178-82.

[41] Thony F, Ferretti G, Sengel C et al. Imaging the abdominal aorta. EMC, Radiodiagnostic-Coeur- poumon, 32-210-C60, 2001, 18 p.

[42] Attlan, Helenon O, Moreau J.F. Sonographic exploration: abdominal aorta. Manuel d'ultrasonologie générale de l'adulte. Masson 1993: 192-193.

[43] Schmidt WA, Kraft H, Vorpahl K, Volker L, Gromnica-Ihle EJ. Color duplex ultrasonography in the diagnosis of temporal arteritis. N Engl J Med 1997; 337: 1336-42.

[44] Schmidt WA, Kraft H, Borkowski A, Gromnica -Ihle EJ. Color duplex ultrasonography in large-vessel giant cell arteritis. Scand J Rheumatol 1999; 28: 374-6

[45] Lauwerys BR, Puttemans T, Houssiau FA, Devogelaer JP. Color Doppler sonography of the temporal arteries in giant cell arteritis and polymialgia rheumatica. J Rheumatol 1997; 24: 1570-4.

[46] Salvarini C, Silingardi M, Ghirarduzzi A, Lo Scocco G, Macchioni P, Bajocchi G, et al. Is duplex ultrasonography useful for the diagnosis of giant-cell arteritis? Ann Intern Med 2002; 137: 232-8.

[47] Christian Agard, Luis said, Thierry Ponge, Jérome Connault, Aghathe Masseau, Marc Antoine pistorius. Frequency of abdominal aortic involvement at the diagnosis of Horton's disease: a study of 20 patients by ultrasound-Doppler and angiomodensitometry. La presse médicale 2009; 38 :11-19.

[48] Baretto SN, Oliveira GH, Michet CJ Jr, Nyman MA, Edwards WD, Kullo IJ. Multiple cardiovascular complications in a patient with relpasing polychondritis. Mayo Clin Proc 2002; 77: 971-4.

[49] Naouli H, Zrihni Y, Jiber H, Bouarhroum A. Abdominal aortic aneurysm revealing Behçet disease. Journal of vascular diseases 2014; 39 (6): 434-438.

[50] Mleyhi S, Ghédira F, Ziadi J, Gara Ali B, Ben Gorbel I, Kaouel K, Ben Mrad M, Denguir R, Kalfat T, Khayati A. Ruptured abdominal subrenal aortic aneurysm inaugural to Takayasu disease in a 39-year-old man. Journal of Vascular Diseases 2013; 38: 373-376.

[51] Chung JW, Kim HC, Choi YH, Kim SJ, Lee W, Park JH. Patterns of aortic involvement in Takayasu arteritis and its clinical implications: evaluation with spiral computed tomography angiography. J Vasc Surg 2007; 45: 906-14.

[52] Salim Chaabouni. Imaging of acquired aortic pathology: about 120 cases. Thesis of medicine year 2012. Faculté de médecine de Sfax.

[53] Navellou J-C, Gil H, Meaux-Ruault N, Magy N, Kantelip B, Dupond J. Inaugural thoracic aortic involvement in Horton's disease. A propos de trois cas. Rev Med interne 2004 ;25 :1416.

[54] Tso E, Flamm SD, White RD, Schvartzman PR, Mascha E, Hoffman GS. Takayasu arteritis: utility and limitations of magnetic resonance imagingi n diagnosis and treatment. Arthritis Rheum 2002; 46: 1634-42.

[55] Pipitone N, Versari A, Salvarani C. Role of imaging studies in the diagnosis and follow-up of large-vessel vasculitis: an update. Rheumatology 2008; 47: 403-8.

[56] Henes JC, Müller M, Krieger J, et al. [18F] FDG-PET/CT as a new and sensitive imaging method for the diagnosis of large vessel vasculitis. Clin Exp Rheumato 2008; 26: S47-52.

[57] Scheel AK, Meller J, Vosshenrich R, et al. Diagnosis and follow up of aortitis in the elderly. Ann Rheum Dis 2004; 63: 1507-10.

[58] Kobayashi Y, Ishii K, Oda K, Nariai T, Tanaka Y, Ishiwata K, et al. Aortic wall inflammation due to Takayasu arteritis imaged with 18F-FDG PET coregistered with enhanced CT. J Nucl Med 2005; 46: 917-22.

[59] Liozon E, Monteil J. Place de la tomographie par émission de positons (TEP) au 18F FDG dans l'exploration des vascularites. Medecine Nucl 2008; 32: 511-22.

[60] Blockmans D. The use of (18F)fluoro-deoxyglucose positron emission tomography in the assessment of large vessel vasculitis. Clin Exp Rheumatol 2003; 21: S15-22.

[61] Mukhtyar C, Guillevin L, Cid MC, et al. EULAR recommendations for the management of large vessel vasculitis. Ann Rheum Dis 2009; 68: 318-23.

[62] Webb M, Chambers A, AL-Nahhas A, Mason JC, Maudlin L, Rahman L et al. The role of 18F-FDGPET in characterising disease activity in Takayasu arteritis. Eur J Nucl Med Mol Imaging 2004; 31:627-34.

[63] Henes JC, Müller M, Krieger J, et al. [18F] FDG-PET/CT as a new and sensitive imaging method for the diagnosis of large vessel vasculitis. Clin Exp Rheumato 2008; 26: S47-52.

[64] Blockmans D, Maes A, Stroobants S, et al. New arguments for a vasculitic nature of polymyalgia rheumatica using positron emission tomography. Rheumatology (Oxford) 1999; 38: 444-7.

[65] Walter MA, Melzer RA, Schindler C, et al. The value of [18F] FDG-PET in the diagnosis of large-vessel vasculitis and the assessment of activity and extent of disease. Eur J Nucl Med Mol Imaging 2005; 32: 674-81.

[66] de Leeuw K, Bijl M, Jager PL. Additional value of positron emission tomography in diagnosis and follow-up of patients with large vessel vasculitides. Clin Exp Rheumatol 2004; 22: S21-6.

[67] Evans JM, O'Fallon WM, Hunder GG. Increased incidence of aortic aneurysm and dissection in giant cell (temporal) arteritis. A population based study. Ann intern Med 1995; 122(7): 502-7

[68] Liu G, Shupak R, Chiu BK. Aortic dissection in giant-cell arteritis. Semin Arthritis Rheum 1995; 25: 160-71.

[69] Blétry O, Aimé P, Degoulet J, Cosserat J, Piette A, Bécour B. Validation of new diagnostic criteria for Takayasu arteritis. Rev Med Interne 1995; 16: 70.

[70] Sharma BK, Jain S, Suri S, Numano F. Diagnostic criteria for Takayasu arteritis. Int J Cardiol 1996; Suppl. 54: S141-7.

[71] Kerr GS, Hallahan CW, Giordano J, Leavitt RY, Fauci AS, Rottem M, et al. Takayasu arteritis. Ann Intern Med 1994; 120: 919-29.

[72] Gene G. Hunder, Daniel A. Bloch, Beat A. Michel, Mary Betty Stevens, William P. Arend. The American College Of Rheumatology 1990 Criteria For The Classification Of Giant Cell Arteritis. Arthritis and Rheumatism, Vol. 33, No. 8 (August 1990).

[73] Vignes S, Vidailhet M, Dormont D et al. Pseudotumoral presentation of Neuro-Behçet: role of Colchicine discontinuation.Rev Med Interne 1998; 19: 55-9.

[74] Hatemi G, Silman A, Bang D et al. Management of Behcet's disease: a systematic literature review for the EULAR evidencebasedrecommendations for the management of Behçet's disease. Ann Rheum Dis 2008; 67: 1656-62.

[75] Huong DLT, Wechsler B, Papo T et al. Arterial lesions in Behcet's disease. J Rheumatol 1995; 22: 2103-13.

[76] Calamia KT, Schirmer M, Melikoglu et al. Major vessel involvement in Behçet disease. Curr Opin Rheumatol 17: 1-8. 2004.

[77] Liang P, Hoffman GS. Advances in the medical and surgical treatment of Takayasu arteritis. Curr Opin Rheumatol 2005; 17: 16-24.

[78] Kieffer E. Surgery of abdominal subrenal aortic aneurysms: surgical techniques. EMC (Elsevier SAS Paris), Techniques chirurgicales-Chirurgie vasculaire-43-154-B, 2005.

[79] Maksimowicz-McKinnon K, Clark TM, Hoffman GS. Limitations of therapy and a guarded prognosis in an American cohort of Takayasu arteritis patients. Arthritis Rheum 2007; 56: 1000-9.

[80] Hoffman GS, Leavitt RY, Kerr GS, Rottem M, Sneller MC, Fauci AS. Treatment of glucocorticoid-resistant or relapsing Takayasu arteritis with methotrexate. Arthritis Rheum 1994; 37: 578-82.

[81] Hoffman GS, Merkel PA, Brasington RD, Lenschow DJ, Liang P. Anti-tumor necrosis factor therapy in patients with difficult-to-treat Takayasu arteritis. Arthritis Rheum 2004; 50: 2296-304.

[82] Sakuma K, Akimoto H, Yokoyama H, et al. Cryopreserved aortic homograft replacement in 3 patients with non-infectious inflammatory vascular disease. J Thorac Cardiovasc Surg 2001; 49: 652-5.

[83] JB Ricco, C. Sessa. Abdominal aorta and iliac artery approaches. Elsevier Masson SAS 2011. 43-034-A

[84] Todd GJ, De Rose JR. Retroperitoneal treatment of inflammatory aortic aneurysms. Ann Chir Vasc 1995; 9: 525-34.

[85] Fabiani JN, Saliou C. Aneurysms of the abdominal subrenal aorta. EMC (Elsevier, Paris), Cardiologie-Angéiologie, 11-645-A-10, 1997, 14p.

[86] Iscan ZH, Vural KM, Bayazit M. Compelling nature of arterial manifestations in Behçet disease. J Vasc Surg 2005; 41: 53-8.

[87] J. Gaudrica, M. Dennerya, C. Jouhanneta, N. Kagana, D. Saadounb, L. Chichea, F. Koskas. Surgical management of inflammatory diseases of the aorta. French National Society of Internal Medicine (SNFMI). Published by Elsevier Masson SAS 2016.

[88] J.P. Becquemin, M. Kirsch, L. Canaud, H. Kobeiter. Surgery of the aortic arch: conventional, endoluminal or hybrid? A strategy à la carte. Revues générales Vasculaire. 2010/10/122.

[89] Kieffer E, Chiche L, Bertal A, Koskas F, Bahnini A, Bla Try O, et al. Descending thoracic and thoraco-abdominal aortic aneurysm in patients with Takayasu's disease. Ann Vasc Surg 2004; 18: 505-13.

[90] Kieffer E, Chiche L, Bertal A, Koskas F, Bahnini A, Blã Try O, et al. Descendingthoracic and thoracoabdominal aortic aneurysm in patients with Takayasu's disease. Ann Vasc Surg 2004; 18: 505-13

[91] Tada Y, Sato O, Ohshima A, Miyata T, Shindo S. Surgical treatment of Takayasu arteritis. Heart Vessels Suppl 1992; 7: 159-67.

[92] Nobuhiro Umehara, Satoshi Saito, Hikaru Ishii, Shigeyuki Aomi, and Hiromi Kurosawa. Rupture of Thoracoabdominal Aortic Aneurysm Associated with Behcet's Disease. Ann Thorac Surg 2007; 84: 1394-6.

[93] Chang-Wei Liu, Wei Ye, Bao Liu, Rong Zeng, Weiwei Wu, and Michael D. Dake, Beijing, China; and Stanford, Calif. Endovascular treatment of aortic pseudoaneurysm in Behçet disease. J Vasc Surg 2009; 50: 1025-30

[94] Inoue K, Hosokawa H, Iwase T et al. Aortic arch reconstruction by transluminally placed endovascular branched stent graft. Circulation, 1999; 100: 316-321.

[95] Tuzun H, Seyahi E, Arslan C, Hamuryudan V, Besirli K, Yazici H. Managementand prognosis of nonpulmonary large arterial disease in patients with Behçet disease. J Vasc Surg 2012; 55: 157-63.

[96] Francis Pesteil, Alessandro Piccardo, Jérémy Tricard, François Bertin, Aurélien Descazeaud, Marc Laskar, Philippe Lacroix.

Inflammatory aneurysms: is endovascular treatment rational? Journal of the French Society of Thoracic and Cardiovascular Surgery June 2016.

[97] Cloatre G, HDA A, Hajji A, Moulay A. Vascular manifestations of Behçet's disease. Médecine et armées 1991, 19, 4, p 199-202.

[98] Kim Y-W, Kim D-I, Park YJ, Yang S-S, Lee G-Y, Kim D-K, et al. Surgical bypass vs endovascular treatment for patients with supra-aortic arterial occlusive disease due to Takayasu arteritis. J Vasc Surg 2012; 55: 693-700.

[99] Kwon TW, Park SJ, Kim HK, Yoon HK, Kim GE, Yu B. Surgical treatment result of abdominal aortic aneurysm in Behçet's disease. Eur J Vasc Endovasc Surg 2008; 35: 173-80.

[100] Sartipy F, Lindström D, Gillgren P, Ternhag A. The role of procalcitonin in Post-implantation Syndrome after EVAR: A Pilot Study. Ann Vasc Surg 2014; 28 (4): 866-73.

[101] Hechelhammer L, Wildermuth S, Lachat ML, Pfammatter T. Endovascular repair of inflammatory abdominal aneurysm: a retrospective analysis of CT follow-up. J Vasc Interv Radiol. 2005; 16(5):737-41.

[102] Tuzun H, Seyahi E, Arslan C, Hamuryudan V, Besirli K, Yazici H. Management and prognosis of non-pulmonary large arterial disease in patients with Behçet disease. J Vasc Surg 2012; 55: 157-63.

[103] T.-W. Kwon, S.-J. Park, H.-K. Kim, H.-K. Yoon, G.-E. Kim and B. Yu. Surgical Treatment Result of Abdominal Aortic Aneurysm in Behc¸et's Disease. Eur J Vasc Endovasc Surg 35, 173-180 (2008) doi:10.1016/j.ejvs.2007.08.013

[104] Bastounis E, Papalambros E, Mermingas V, Maltezos CH, Diamantis T, Balas P. Secondary aortoduodenal fistulae. J Cardiovasc Surg 1997; 38: 457-564.

[105] H. Z. Iscan, M. K. Gol, N. Erdol, L. K. Yildiz, M. Bayazit and O. Tasdemir. Behçet's Aortitis - a Case Report: False Aneurysm Rupture and Aortico-duodenal Fistula. EJVES Extra 1, 21-23 (2001).

[106] Isobe M. Takayasu arteritis revisited: current diagnosis and treatment. Int J Cardiol 2013; 168: 3-10.

[107] Paravastu SCV, Ghosh J, Murray D, Farquharson FG, Serracino-Inglott F, Walker MG. A systematic review of open versus endovascular repair of inflammatory abdominal aortic aneurysms. Eur J Vasc Endovasc Surg 2009; 38(3): 291-7.

[108] Puchner S, Bucek RA, Loewe C et al. Endovascular repair of inflammatory aortic aneurysms: long-term results. AJR. 2006; 186(4): 1144-7.

[109] Van Bommel EFH, Van der Veer SJ, Hendrikksz, Bleumink GS. Persistent chronic peri-aortitis (inflammatory aneurysm) after abdominal aortic aneurysm repair: systematic review of the literature. Vasc Med 2008 ; 13: 293-303.

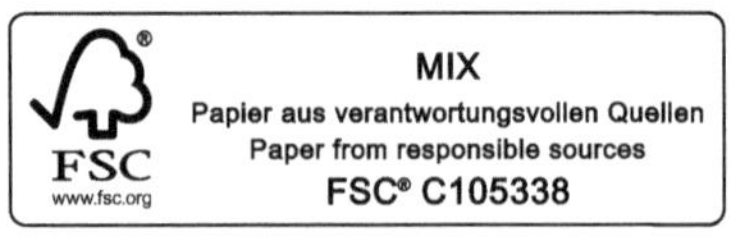

Printed by Books on Demand GmbH, Norderstedt / Germany